JUST PLANE yoga

doing it in tight places

Trish A. McCarty

Trish McCarty

Published by StarShine Press
www.starshinepress.com

First edition, 2012

ISBN: 0982613393
ISBN-13: 9780982613399

THIS BOOK IS DEDICATED TO:

One of my best Yoga teachers; Sandra Summerfield Kozak continuously encouraged me as I developed as a Yoga teacher and a banker, many times helping me to understand the balance. She also taught me the importance of practicing Pranayama as one of the profound effects on my life.

I also want to dedicate this to all of the students, teachers, volunteers and partners of StarShine Academy schools. StarShine has given to me the greatest Yoga experience.

CONTENTS

	Acknowledgments	i
1	Before You Begin	5
2	Yoga	9
3	Take a Deep Breath	11
4	Asana #1	13
5	Asana #2	16
6	Asana #3	17
7	Asana #4	18
8	Asana #5	19
9	Asana #6	20
10	Asana #7	22

ACKNOWLEDGMENTS

I extend my appreciation and thanks to the many Yoga teachers I have had in my life. Many of you did not know you were my teacher and some of you did not know anything about Yoga, and yet you influenced my learning. My Mother, Ruby Sanders gave me the most encouragement and continues to on a daily basis. My first Yoga teacher was on television, *Lilias Folan for Yoga*; one of the most breakthrough television programs at the time. She taught me that gentle Yoga is a wonderful approach. My next teacher was one of the first Iyengar Certified teachers in the United States. After a two-year intensive certification program, she said she would not certify me unless I promised to teach and share Yoga at least once a week for the rest of my life. So I promised, even though teaching was not why I wanted to know Yoga; it was for my own knowledge. I learned though, that good information is made to share. Little did I know at the time, how much this would influence my life as an executive and an entrepreneur, eventually to dedicate my life to establishing schools for all children based on learning about body, mind and spirit along with academics, as founder of StarShine Academy International Schools.

I have had many amazing teachers and I thank you all, especially Sandra. And I thank the Phoenician Resort Spa for letting me share my Yoga for so many years with so many needy travelers who asked me to publish this book.

JUST   PLANE YOGA

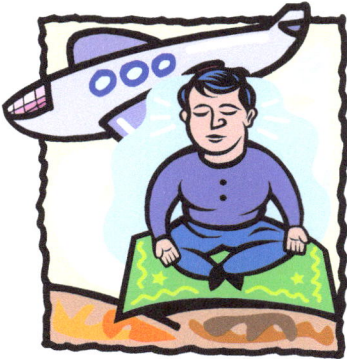

...doing it

in tight places

♥

everywhere

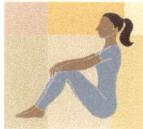

Trish McCarty

Trish McCarty

Before you begin

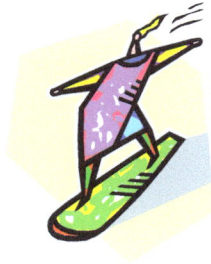

Wear **plane** clothes. Fancy ones (or blue jeans) restrict movement and aren't you usually squished into a tight spot on a **plane** anyway? But if you must wear a suit and tie--loosen it up, and still do **plane yoga**. Keep some water close by, and drink it often.

It's nice to create some atmosphere when you do **yoga**, whether on a **plane**, a hotel room, or at home. Incense on a plane is not going to work, but there are other ways to use the powerful mood enhancer of smell. Carry a small inhaler with your favorite scent of aromatherapy. Lavender oil is for sale in most grocery stores and the smell is usually relaxing. Eucalyptus is another favorite. Aromatherapy oils might be healthier than smelling perfume.

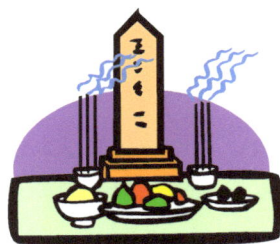

Listening to calming music is a great mood enhancer and using earphones helps to block the noise of the **plane**.

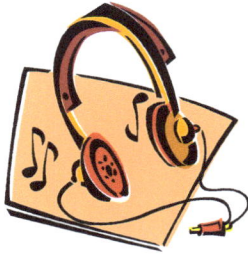

I usually listen to harp music or Native American flute music like Carlos Nakai. Pandora labels it New Age Music or Zen Music.

I know, many of you are perfectionists and want to do everything exactly as directed but that's not Yoga. Yoga is about you. Don't worry if you get out of order--go ahead and skip to number 6. You won't have anybody tell you you're not good enough. Yoga is always about being better.

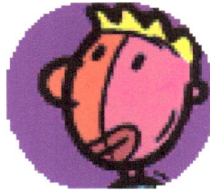

Now you're ready. You're headset is on, you've smelled your aromatherapy oil and you're pretty comfortable in your relaxed clothes.

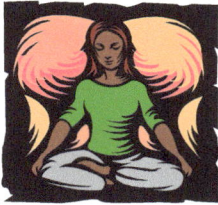

Yoga comes from the same word as yoke, and it means to "yoke" your body together = **body+mind+spirit.** Awareness of yourself begins with noticing breath, or life force, called "Pranayama" in Sanskrit. Concentrating on your breath immediately harnesses your brain, your thoughts. The more you practice concentrating on your breathing, the easier it gets and the less mind clutter you will have. Runaway (or runway) thoughts can be quieted with **plane** breathing exercises.

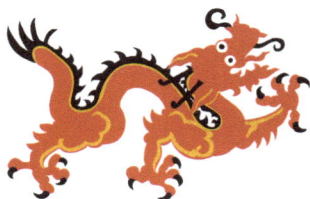

1 2 3 4 5 6

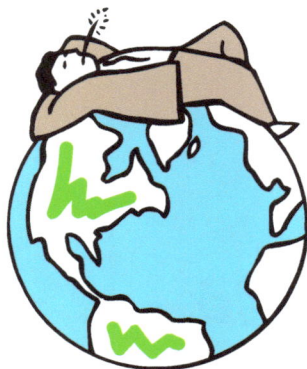

1 2 3

Put your seat back and begin by lightly closing your eyes. Take a slow even breath in through your nose to a count of six... 1 2 3 4 5 6. Try to feel the air go across the back of your throat...it helps to relax. Feel your lungs expand. Soften your belly. Hold your breath for the count of three 1 2 3. And then with a steady rhythm, begin to exhale through your nose (if you can) and count all the way through to 12. 1 2 3 4 5 6 7 8 9 10 11 12 . Hold again for three before you breathe in again. 1 2 3. During the holds, the most happens, so try to do it.

Take a deep breath...

BREATHE IN (NOSE) 1 2 3 4 5 6

HOLD 1 2 3

BREATHE OUT (NOSE) 1 2 3 4 5 6 7 8 9 10 11 12

HOLD 1 2 3   Repeat...

Do this exercise for 3-20 minutes, each time trying to go a little longer. It will do wonders for your heart and lungs. Your whole body will love it after just a few minutes. The calming and clearer thinking can last for hours when you do this breathing exercise for 20 minutes or more. You might want to start everyday with this breathing exercise at home. Do this exercise before you start your **Plane Yoga** each time. Your muscles will work better when they have been pumped with a bunch of oxygen. Plus, it will keep your body more relaxed and fluid. (It also makes the skin on your face look better.)

(If you aren't on a plane, try these exercises while sitting on an exercise ball...it will increase the intensity of the exercises.)

Trish McCarty

♥Asana Exercise #1

Put both feet flat on the floor, about hip distance apart. Put your hands on your lap, palms up. Sit tall. Picture your spine beginning at your tailbone reaching to the ceiling, 1 vertebra at a time, one on top of the other. The top of your head reaching as high as possible while remaining seated. Take two more breaths, just like the beginning:

IN 1 2 3 4 5 6 , HOLD 1 2 3 , OUT 1 2 3 4 5 6 7 8 9 10 11 12 HOLD 1 2 3 Repeat...

While sitting tall, bend right ear toward the right shoulder, while you keep both shoulders down.

Hold and Breathe S.l.o.w IN 1 2 3 4 , OUT 1 2 3 4 IN 1 2 3 4 , OUT 1 2 3 4. Each time you exhale try to relax the other side of your neck. Keep shoulders down and back sitting up straight. Take a deep breath and

s lo w l y return your head to the center.

Now, bend left ear toward the left shoulder. Again, keep back straight and shoulders down. Repeat breathing pattern.

Hold and Breathe S.l.o.w IN 1 2 3 4 , OUT 1 2 3 4 IN 1 2 3 4 , OUT 1 2 3 4. Each time you exhale try to relax the other side of your neck. Keep shoulders down and back sitting up straight. Take a deep breath and

s lo w l y return your head to the center.

Now bring chin to your chest...Repeat breathing pattern.

Hold and Breathe S.l.o.w IN 1 2 3 4 , OUT 1 2 3 4 IN 1 2 3 4 , OUT 1 2 3 4. Each time you exhale try to relax the other side of your neck. Keep shoulders down and back sitting up straight. Take a deep breath and

s lo w l y return your head to the center.

Finally, bring chin toward the ceiling, back straight, shoulders down. Repeat breathing.

You should do this at your office at least every 45 minutes of working at your desk.

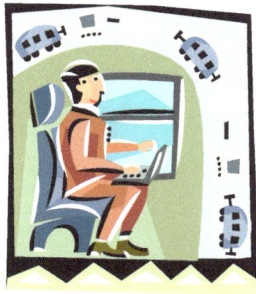

♥Asana Exercise # 2

Lift right hand, bring to outside of left lap, hold side of your leg, keeping feet on floor and back straight, begin to twist slightly toward the left.. As you begin to twist, try to start the twist from your tailbone, one vertebra at a time all the way up to your head, looking over your left shoulder...you can close your eyes if you don't   want   to   stare   at   your neighbor...BREATHE...hold for at least four 1 2 3 4 and then S LO W L Y unwind. Release your right hand and change to other side. Lift left hand and hold outside of right leg, next to lap. Twist slowly toward the right, one vertebra at a time, tailbone first, all the way   up   to   your   head,   look   over   your   right shoulder....BREATHE...hold for at least four 1 2 3 4 .

UNWIND ...S L O W L Y...

♥Asana Exercise #3

With each hand hold on to your legs on either side of your lap. As you sit tall, begin to arch your back into your seat, rolling each vertebra back starting with your tailbone and ending with your forehead pointing toward your belly button. Roll your shoulders forward...again hold at least for four

1 2 3 4 and BREATHE. As you move into the opposite exercise, you will arch your back, tailbone first, away from the seat, one vertebra at a time, chest out as far from the seat as the top of your head tilts back toward the rear. HOLD for 1 2 3 4. This is a nice one to repeat   These exercises loosen your back, which most of us need desperately. Back pain is responsible for most of missed workdays...AND the way you hold your back is the first sign of age, unless you do PLANE YOGA...

♥Asana Exercise # 4

A little twist to the twist... Cross left leg over right leg...do what you can with your space allotment. Grab the outside of your left thigh with your right hand. Twist toward the left, starting with your tailbone, all the way up to your head, looking again over your left shoulder. BREATHE...HOLD 1 2 3 4 . Unwind slowly. Change legs...right over the left. Reach across with your left hand and slowly twist around toward the right...one vertebra at a time...BREATHE...HOLD 1 2 3 4 . Unwind slowly. Relax your face.

♥Asana Exercise # 5

Feet flat on the floor, hip distance apart. Back straight, top of your head reaching up toward the ceiling. Interlock fingers, press palms away from your body--you may not have enough room to extend your arms forward in front of you, but try...BREATHE...Then INHALE, raise your arms over your head, keeping palms outward until your arms are next to your ears and straight up, palms facing the ceiling....*Now I know, you feel conspicuous, go ahead anyway...be the leader, they all need the same thing, and even if they don't do it----you'll be the one feeling good---they'll wish that they had...*

This exercise gets your heart pumping so it is really good for you when you are cooped up for hours. It will help the blood to flow and it feels great.

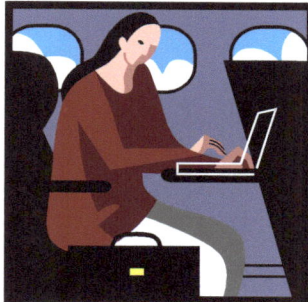

♥Asana Exercise # 6

Keeping back straight, raise each knee toward chest----do what you can. Then put both feet flat on the floor, hands resting on your knees, palms down. Tighten all muscles in your calves, thighs, stomach and hip area---as tight as you can, try to lift yourself a little off of your seat--no help from your hands--only using your feet, stomach and leg/hip muscles. Keep BREATHING but hold the position as long and tight as you can. This will also get the blood flowing and is a great way to strengthen the muscles. Repeat this exercise at least 5 times. You will feel like falling asleep after this one, but stay with it, you're almost done.

You've worked hard and it is going to soooooo pay off-- you'll be ready to party when you get off of the plane because you did your own *Just Plane Yoga* and re-energized yourself while everybody else will wish they knew what you know.

♥Asana Exercise # 7

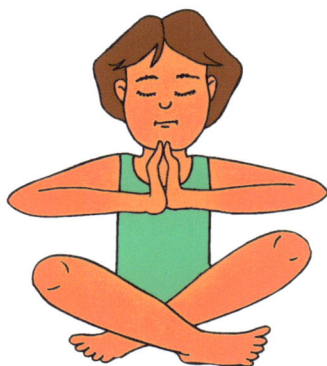

Ok---last one---press your palms together (remember the old isometric exercises) --keep even pressure as you make three circles toward the right.

1. Start pressing with your palms in front of your chest
2. Move your pressed palms upward toward your forehead--higher if you can.
3. Start to make a slow circle toward the right as you bring your palms down
4. Press them in a circle coming in front of your belly button and keep making a circle.
5. Repeat three times while continuing to press together.
6. Then without letting the pressure off, bring palms back to the front of your chest.
7. Repeat three times toward the left.
8. As the arms rise--breathe in through the nose.
9. As the arms move down, exhale through the nose.

As you begin to do these exercises on a daily basis and for sure when you travel, you will be absolutely amazed at how you look and feel. People around you will comment on the extra energy you seem to have, and how much happier you look.

Be thankful for the uniqueness of who you are and look for the unique way that you can contribute to make the world and your life better and then do it. You are the only one like you. We need your uniqueness. The world needs you.

Namaste'

Love ♥ Peace,

TRISH A

ABOUT THE AUTHOR

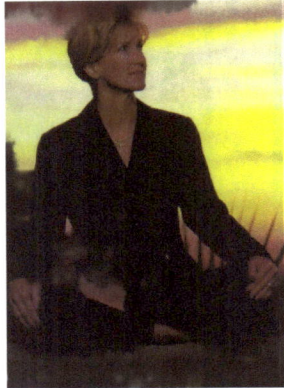

Trish A. McCarty has been a student of Yoga since age 17. At 20, she was certified in the BKS Iyengar method of Yoga practice while living in San Diego, California, with a promise to teach yoga at least once a week for the rest of her life. She has a deep commitment to learning and teaching Pranayama.

Her Yoga practice and teaching sustained her through a very competitive, successful career in business and banking and opening a school in 2002 for high-risk children, StarShine Academy.org. She attributes her success in business as a direct result of understanding the power of practicing body, mind, spirit, health, wealth and happiness in every moment.

She has taught in resorts around the world and has been a Yoga teacher at the 5-star internationally known, Phoenician Resort Wellness Center in Phoenix, Arizona since the resort opened in 1989, until last year when she left to pursue a greater impact through establishing StarShine schools and spend more time writing and speaking to larger audiences about education and integrating body, mind, spirit, health, wealth and happiness, as a means to peace.

Trish has said for years, that if everyone did Yoga as exercise and health maintenance , the world and its inhabitants would be at peace.

To download free exercises and information go to:
www.JustPlaneYoga.com

www.ingramcontent.com/pod-product-compliance
Lightning Source LLC
Chambersburg PA
CBHW041303290326
41931CB00032B/36